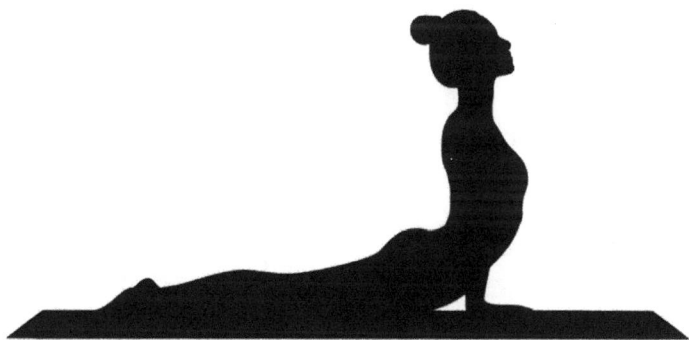

Belongs To

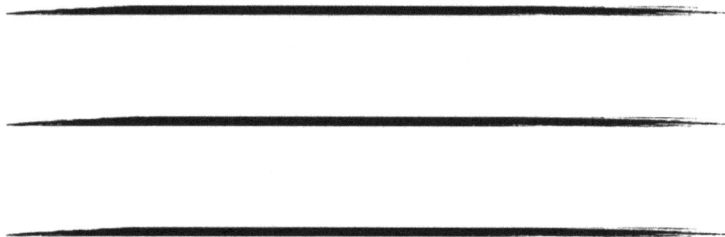

BODY MEASUREMENT

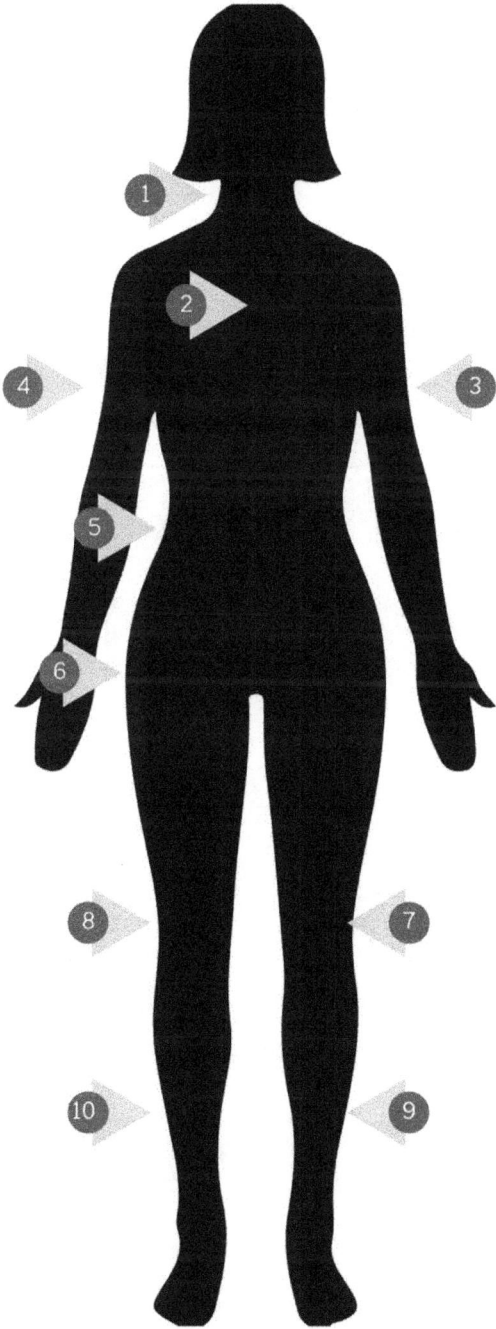

BEFORE		
DATE:		
WEIGHT:		
1	NECK	
2	CHEST	
3	LEFT ARM	
4	RIGHT ARM	
5	WAIST	
6	HIPS	
7	LEFT THIGH	
8	RIGHT THIGH	
9	LEFT CALF:	
10	RIGHT CALF	

MY FITNESS GOAL

5 Reasons I want to get healthier.

1.

2.

3.

4.

5.

SHORT TERM GOALS	LONG TERM GOALS

NOTE TO SELF

ACTION PLANS

REWARD

REQUIRED CHANGES

HABITS I NEED TO CHANGE

FRIDGE SETTING

ROOM SETTING

TRIGGERS

COPPING METHODS

NOTES

30-Days
Challenge

30-Days
Challenge

30-Days
Challenge

MONTHLY TRACKER

MONTH 1: _____

WEEK 1	WEEK 2	WEEK 3	WEEK 4

MONTH 2: _____

WEEK 1	WEEK 2	WEEK 3	WEEK 4

MONTH 3: _____

WEEK 1	WEEK 2	WEEK 3	WEEK 4

NOTES	BEFORE	AFTER

TARGET WEIGHT

DATE: /   /   S   M   T   W   T   F   S

MY DAILY GOALS

MY MOTIVATION

WATER TRACKER

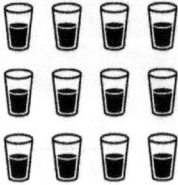

MEALS AND SNACKS

BREAKFAST	LUNCH	DINNER	SNACKS

EXERCISE	REPS	SET -1	SET -2	SET -3	NOTE

TODAY'S FEELINGS	FEELINGS I WANT TO FEEL TOMORROW

DATE: /   /   S   M   T   W   T   F   S

MY DAILY GOALS

MY MOTIVATION

WATER TRACKER

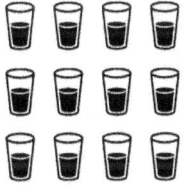

MEALS AND SNACKS

BREAKFAST	LUNCH	DINNER	SNACKS

EXERCISE	REPS	SET -1	SET -2	SET -3	NOTE

TODAY'S FEELINGS	FEELINGS I WANT TO FEEL TOMORROW

DATE: /   /   S   M   T   W   T   F   S

MY DAILY GOALS

MY MOTIVATION

WATER TRACKER

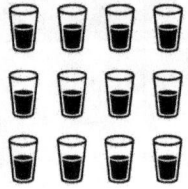

MEALS AND SNACKS

BREAKFAST	LUNCH	DINNER	SNACKS

EXERCISE	REPS	SET -1	SET -2	SET -3	NOTE

TODAY'S FEELINGS	FEELINGS I WANT TO FEEL TOMORROW

DATE: / / S M T W T F S

MY DAILY GOALS

WATER
TRACKER

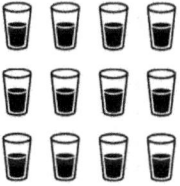

MEALS AND SNACKS

BREAKFAST	LUNCH	DINNER	SNACKS

EXERCISE	REPS	SET -1	SET -2	SET -3	NOTE

TODAY'S FEELINGS	FEELINGS I WANT TO FEEL TOMORROW

DATE: /   /   S   M   T   W   T   F   S

MY DAILY GOALS

MY MOTIVATION

WATER TRACKER

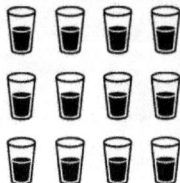

MEALS AND SNACKS

BREAKFAST	LUNCH	DINNER	SNACKS

EXERCISE	REPS	SET -1	SET -2	SET -3	NOTE

TODAY'S FEELINGS	FEELINGS I WANT TO FEEL TOMORROW

DATE: / /   S M T W T F S

MY DAILY GOALS

MY MOTIVATION

WATER TRACKER

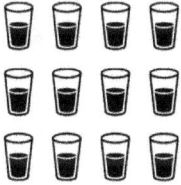

MEALS AND SNACKS

Breakfast	Lunch	Dinner	Snacks

Exercise	Reps	Set -1	Set -2	Set -3	Note

TODAY'S FEELINGS	FEELINGS I WANT TO FEEL TOMORROW

DATE: /   /   S   M   T   W   T   F   S

MY DAILY GOALS

MY MOTIVATION

WATER TRACKER

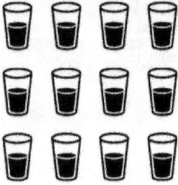

MEALS AND SNACKS

BREAKFAST	LUNCH	DINNER	SNACKS

EXERCISE	REPS	SET -1	SET -2	SET -3	NOTE

TODAY'S FEELINGS	FEELINGS I WANT TO FEEL TOMORROW

DATE: /   /   S   M   T   W   T   F   S

MY DAILY GOALS

MY MOTIVATION

WATER TRACKER

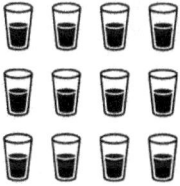

MEALS AND SNACKS

BREAKFAST	LUNCH	DINNER	SNACKS

EXERCISE	REPS	SET -1	SET -2	SET -3	NOTE

TODAY'S FEELINGS	FEELINGS I WANT TO FEEL TOMORROW

DATE: /   /   S   M   T   W   T   F   S

MY DAILY GOALS

WATER
TRACKER

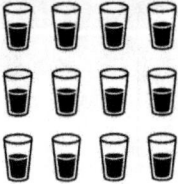

MEALS AND SNACKS

BREAKFAST	LUNCH	DINNER	SNACKS

EXERCISE	REPS	SET -1	SET -2	SET -3	NOTE

TODAY'S FEELINGS	FEELINGS I WANT TO FEEL TOMORROW

DATE: /   /   S   M   T   W   T   F   S

MY DAILY GOALS

MY MOTIVATION

WATER TRACKER

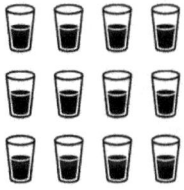

MEALS AND SNACKS

BREAKFAST	LUNCH	DINNER	SNACKS

EXERCISE	REPS	SET -1	SET -2	SET -3	NOTE

TODAY'S FEELINGS	FEELINGS I WANT TO FEEL TOMORROW

DATE: /   /   S   M   T   W   T   F   S

MY DAILY GOALS

MY MOTIVATION

WATER
TRACKER

MEALS AND SNACKS

BREAKFAST	LUNCH	DINNER	SNACKS

EXERCISE	REPS	SET -1	SET -2	SET -3	NOTE

TODAY'S FEELINGS	FEELINGS I WANT TO FEEL TOMORROW

DATE: /   /   S M T W T F S

MY DAILY GOALS

MY MOTIVATION

WATER TRACKER

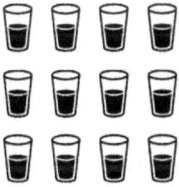

MEALS AND SNACKS

BREAKFAST	LUNCH	DINNER	SNACKS

EXERCISE	REPS	SET -1	SET -2	SET -3	NOTE

TODAY'S FEELINGS

FEELINGS I WANT TO FEEL TOMORROW

DATE: /   /   S   M   T   W   T   F   S

MY DAILY GOALS

MY MOTIVATION

WATER TRACKER

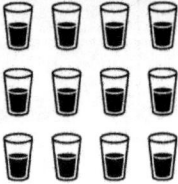

MEALS AND SNACKS

BREAKFAST	LUNCH	DINNER	SNACKS

EXERCISE	REPS	SET -1	SET -2	SET -3	NOTE

TODAY'S FEELINGS	FEELINGS I WANT TO FEEL TOMORROW

DATE: /   /   S   M   T   W   T   F   S

MY DAILY GOALS

MY MOTIVATION

WATER TRACKER

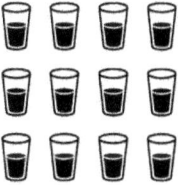

MEALS AND SNACKS

BREAKFAST	LUNCH	DINNER	SNACKS

EXERCISE	REPS	SET -1	SET -2	SET -3	NOTE

TODAY'S FEELINGS	FEELINGS I WANT TO FEEL TOMORROW

DATE: /   /   S   M   T   W   T   F   S

MY DAILY GOALS

MY MOTIVATION

WATER TRACKER

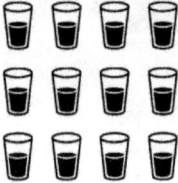

MEALS AND SNACKS

BREAKFAST	LUNCH	DINNER	SNACKS

EXERCISE	REPS	SET -1	SET -2	SET -3	NOTE

TODAY'S FEELINGS	FEELINGS I WANT TO FEEL TOMORROW

DATE: /   /   S   M   T   W   T   F   S

MY DAILY GOALS

MY MOTIVATION

WATER TRACKER

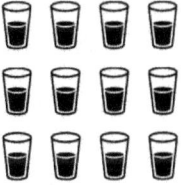

MEALS AND SNACKS

BREAKFAST	LUNCH	DINNER	SNACKS

EXERCISE	REPS	SET -1	SET -2	SET -3	NOTE

TODAY'S FEELINGS	FEELINGS I WANT TO FEEL TOMORROW

DATE: /   /   S   M   T   W   T   F   S

MY DAILY GOALS

MY MOTIVATION

WATER TRACKER

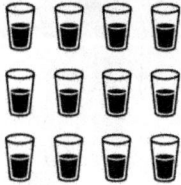

MEALS AND SNACKS

BREAKFAST	LUNCH	DINNER	SNACKS

EXERCISE	REPS	SET -1	SET -2	SET -3	NOTE

TODAY'S FEELINGS	FEELINGS I WANT TO FEEL TOMORROW

DATE: / /   S   M   T   W   T   F   S

MY DAILY GOALS

MY MOTIVATION

WATER
TRACKER

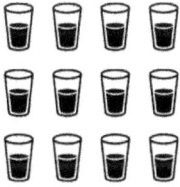

MEALS AND SNACKS

BREAKFAST	LUNCH	DINNER	SNACKS

EXERCISE	REPS	SET -1	SET -2	SET -3	NOTE

TODAY'S FEELINGS	FEELINGS I WANT TO FEEL TOMORROW

DATE: /   /   S   M   T   W   T   F   S

MY DAILY GOALS

WATER
TRACKER

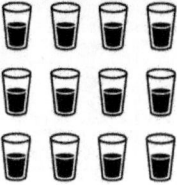

MEALS AND SNACKS

BREAKFAST	LUNCH	DINNER	SNACKS

EXERCISE	REPS	SET -1	SET -2	SET -3	NOTE

TODAY'S FEELINGS

FEELINGS I WANT TO
FEEL TOMORROW

DATE: /   /   S   M   T   W   T   F   S

MY DAILY GOALS

MY MOTIVATION

WATER TRACKER

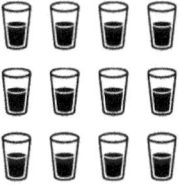

MEALS AND SNACKS

BREAKFAST	LUNCH	DINNER	SNACKS

EXERCISE	REPS	SET -1	SET -2	SET -3	NOTE

TODAY'S FEELINGS	FEELINGS I WANT TO FEEL TOMORROW

DATE: /   /   S   M   T   W   T   F   S

MY DAILY GOALS

MY MOTIVATION

WATER TRACKER

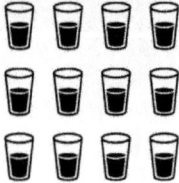

MEALS AND SNACKS

BREAKFAST	LUNCH	DINNER	SNACKS

EXERCISE	REPS	SET -1	SET -2	SET -3	NOTE

TODAY'S FEELINGS

FEELINGS I WANT TO FEEL TOMORROW

DATE: /   /   S   M   T   W   T   F   S

MY DAILY GOALS

MY MOTIVATION

WATER TRACKER

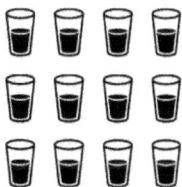

MEALS AND SNACKS

BREAKFAST	LUNCH	DINNER	SNACKS

EXERCISE	REPS	SET -1	SET -2	SET -3	NOTE

TODAY'S FEELINGS	FEELINGS I WANT TO FEEL TOMORROW

DATE: /   /   S   M   T   W   T   F   S

MY DAILY GOALS

WATER TRACKER

MEALS AND SNACKS

BREAKFAST	LUNCH	DINNER	SNACKS

EXERCISE	REPS	SET -1	SET -2	SET -3	NOTE

TODAY'S FEELINGS	FEELINGS I WANT TO FEEL TOMORROW

DATE: / /   S M T W T F S

MY DAILY GOALS

MY MOTIVATION

WATER TRACKER

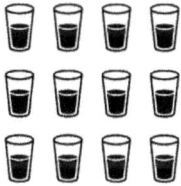

MEALS AND SNACKS

BREAKFAST	LUNCH	DINNER	SNACKS

EXERCISE	REPS	SET -1	SET -2	SET -3	NOTE

TODAY'S FEELINGS	FEELINGS I WANT TO FEEL TOMORROW

DATE: /   /   S   M   T   W   T   F   S

MY DAILY GOALS

MY MOTIVATION

WATER TRACKER

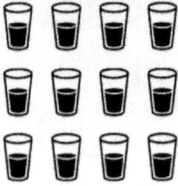

MEALS AND SNACKS

BREAKFAST	LUNCH	DINNER	SNACKS

EXERCISE	REPS	SET -1	SET -2	SET -3	NOTE

TODAY'S FEELINGS	FEELINGS I WANT TO FEEL TOMORROW

DATE: / /   S   M   T   W   T   F   S

MY DAILY GOALS

MY MOTIVATION

WATER TRACKER

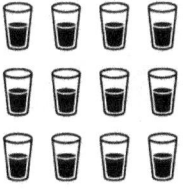

MEALS AND SNACKS

BREAKFAST	LUNCH	DINNER	SNACKS

EXERCISE	REPS	SET -1	SET -2	SET -3	NOTE

TODAY'S FEELINGS	FEELINGS I WANT TO FEEL TOMORROW

DATE: /   /   S   M   T   W   T   F   S

MY DAILY GOALS

MY MOTIVATION

WATER TRACKER

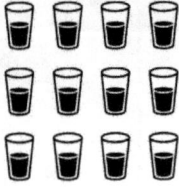

MEALS AND SNACKS

BREAKFAST	LUNCH	DINNER	SNACKS

EXERCISE	REPS	SET -1	SET -2	SET -3	NOTE

TODAY'S FEELINGS	FEELINGS I WANT TO FEEL TOMORROW

DATE: /   /   S   M   T   W   T   F   S

MY DAILY GOALS

MY MOTIVATION

WATER TRACKER

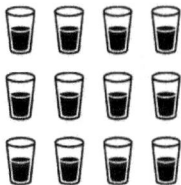

MEALS AND SNACKS

BREAKFAST	LUNCH	DINNER	SNACKS

EXERCISE	REPS	SET -1	SET -2	SET -3	NOTE

TODAY'S FEELINGS	FEELINGS I WANT TO FEEL TOMORROW

DATE: ___ / ___ / ___   S   M   T   W   T   F   S

MY DAILY GOALS

WATER TRACKER

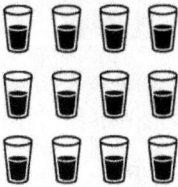

MEALS AND SNACKS

BREAKFAST	LUNCH	DINNER	SNACKS

EXERCISE	REPS	SET -1	SET -2	SET -3	NOTE

TODAY'S FEELINGS	FEELINGS I WANT TO FEEL TOMORROW

DATE: / /   S   M   T   W   T   F   S

MY DAILY GOALS

WATER TRACKER

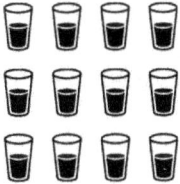

MEALS AND SNACKS

Breakfast	Lunch	Dinner	Snacks

Exercise	Reps	Set -1	Set -2	Set -3	Note

TODAY'S FEELINGS

FEELINGS I WANT TO FEEL TOMORROW

DATE: / /   S   M   T   W   T   F   S

MY DAILY GOALS

MY MOTIVATION

WATER TRACKER

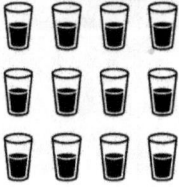

MEALS AND SNACKS

BREAKFAST	LUNCH	DINNER	SNACKS

EXERCISE	REPS	SET -1	SET -2	SET -3	NOTE

TODAY'S FEELINGS	FEELINGS I WANT TO FEEL TOMORROW

DATE: /   /   S   M   T   W   T   F   S

MY DAILY GOALS

MY MOTIVATION

WATER TRACKER

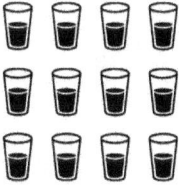

MEALS AND SNACKS

BREAKFAST	LUNCH	DINNER	SNACKS

EXERCISE	REPS	SET -1	SET -2	SET -3	NOTE

TODAY'S FEELINGS

FEELINGS I WANT TO FEEL TOMORROW

DATE: /   /   S   M   T   W   T   F   S

MY DAILY GOALS

MY MOTIVATION

WATER TRACKER

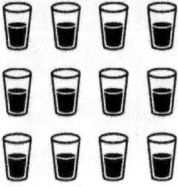

MEALS AND SNACKS

BREAKFAST	LUNCH	DINNER	SNACKS

EXERCISE	REPS	SET -1	SET -2	SET -3	NOTE

TODAY'S FEELINGS	FEELINGS I WANT TO FEEL TOMORROW

DATE: /   /   S   M   T   W   T   F   S

MY DAILY GOALS

MY MOTIVATION

WATER TRACKER

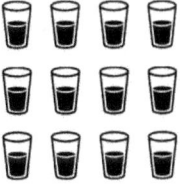

MEALS AND SNACKS

BREAKFAST	LUNCH	DINNER	SNACKS

EXERCISE	REPS	SET -1	SET -2	SET -3	NOTE

TODAY'S FEELINGS	FEELINGS I WANT TO FEEL TOMORROW

DATE: /   /   S   M   T   W   T   F   S

MY DAILY GOALS

WATER
TRACKER

MEALS AND SNACKS

BREAKFAST	LUNCH	DINNER	SNACKS

EXERCISE	REPS	SET -1	SET -2	SET -3	NOTE

TODAY'S FEELINGS	FEELINGS I WANT TO FEEL TOMORROW

DATE: /   /   S   M   T   W   T   F   S

MY DAILY GOALS

WATER TRACKER

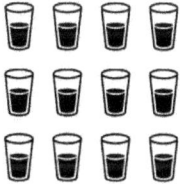

MEALS AND SNACKS

BREAKFAST	LUNCH	DINNER	SNACKS

EXERCISE	REPS	SET -1	SET -2	SET -3	NOTE

TODAY'S FEELINGS	FEELINGS I WANT TO FEEL TOMORROW

DATE: /   /   S   M   T   W   T   F   S

MY DAILY GOALS

MY MOTIVATION

WATER TRACKER

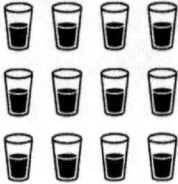

MEALS AND SNACKS

BREAKFAST	LUNCH	DINNER	SNACKS

EXERCISE	REPS	SET -1	SET -2	SET -3	NOTE

TODAY'S FEELINGS	FEELINGS I WANT TO FEEL TOMORROW

DATE: / /   S M T W T F S

MY DAILY GOALS

MY MOTIVATION

WATER TRACKER

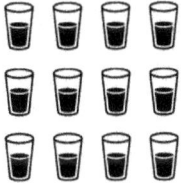

MEALS AND SNACKS

Breakfast	Lunch	Dinner	Snacks

Exercise	Reps	Set -1	Set -2	Set -3	Note

TODAY'S FEELINGS

FEELINGS I WANT TO FEEL TOMORROW

DATE: /   /   S   M   T   W   T   F   S

MY DAILY GOALS

MY MOTIVATION

WATER
TRACKER

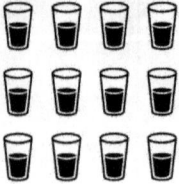

MEALS AND SNACKS

BREAKFAST	LUNCH	DINNER	SNACKS

EXERCISE	REPS	SET -1	SET -2	SET -3	NOTE

TODAY'S FEELINGS	FEELINGS I WANT TO FEEL TOMORROW

DATE: /   /   S   M   T   W   T   F   S

MY DAILY GOALS

MY MOTIVATION

WATER TRACKER

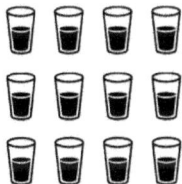

MEALS AND SNACKS

BREAKFAST	LUNCH	DINNER	SNACKS

EXERCISE	REPS	SET -1	SET -2	SET -3	NOTE

TODAY'S FEELINGS	FEELINGS I WANT TO FEEL TOMORROW

DATE: /   /   S   M   T   W   T   F   S

MY DAILY GOALS

WATER
TRACKER

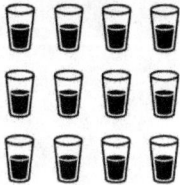

MEALS AND SNACKS

BREAKFAST	LUNCH	DINNER	SNACKS

EXERCISE	REPS	SET -1	SET -2	SET -3	NOTE

TODAY'S FEELINGS	FEELINGS I WANT TO FEEL TOMORROW

DATE: /   /   S   M   T   W   T   F   S

MY DAILY GOALS

MY MOTIVATION

WATER
TRACKER

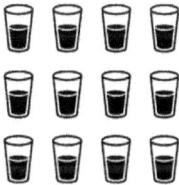

MEALS AND SNACKS

BREAKFAST	LUNCH	DINNER	SNACKS

EXERCISE	REPS	SET -1	SET -2	SET -3	NOTE

TODAY'S FEELINGS

FEELINGS I WANT TO
FEEL TOMORROW

DATE: /   /   S   M   T   W   T   F   S

MY DAILY GOALS

WATER
TRACKER

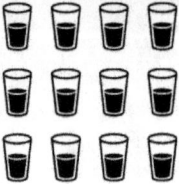

MEALS AND SNACKS

BREAKFAST	LUNCH	DINNER	SNACKS

EXERCISE	REPS	SET -1	SET -2	SET -3	NOTE

TODAY'S FEELINGS	FEELINGS I WANT TO FEEL TOMORROW

DATE: /   /   S   M   T   W   T   F   S

MY DAILY GOALS

WATER
TRACKER

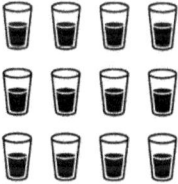

MEALS AND SNACKS

BREAKFAST	LUNCH	DINNER	SNACKS

EXERCISE	REPS	SET -1	SET -2	SET -3	NOTE

TODAY'S FEELINGS	FEELINGS I WANT TO FEEL TOMORROW

DATE: / / S M T W T F S

MY DAILY GOALS

MY MOTIVATION

WATER TRACKER

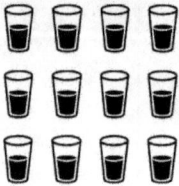

MEALS AND SNACKS

BREAKFAST	LUNCH	DINNER	SNACKS

EXERCISE	REPS	SET -1	SET -2	SET -3	NOTE

TODAY'S FEELINGS

FEELINGS I WANT TO FEEL TOMORROW

DATE: / /   S M T W T F S

MY DAILY GOALS

MY MOTIVATION

WATER TRACKER

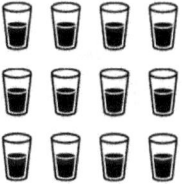

MEALS AND SNACKS

BREAKFAST	LUNCH	DINNER	SNACKS

EXERCISE	REPS	SET -1	SET -2	SET -3	NOTE

TODAY'S FEELINGS	FEELINGS I WANT TO FEEL TOMORROW

DATE: /   /   S   M   T   W   T   F   S

MY DAILY GOALS

MY MOTIVATION

WATER TRACKER

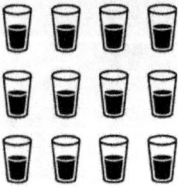

MEALS AND SNACKS

BREAKFAST	LUNCH	DINNER	SNACKS

EXERCISE	REPS	SET -1	SET -2	SET -3	NOTE

TODAY'S FEELINGS	FEELINGS I WANT TO FEEL TOMORROW

DATE: /   /   S   M   T   W   T   F   S

MY DAILY GOALS

MY MOTIVATION

WATER TRACKER

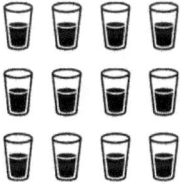

MEALS AND SNACKS

BREAKFAST	LUNCH	DINNER	SNACKS

EXERCISE	REPS	SET -1	SET -2	SET -3	NOTE

TODAY'S FEELINGS	FEELINGS I WANT TO FEEL TOMORROW

DATE: /   /   S   M   T   W   T   F   S

MY DAILY GOALS

MY MOTIVATION

WATER
TRACKER

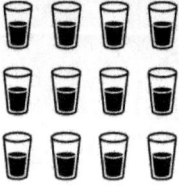

MEALS AND SNACKS

BREAKFAST	LUNCH	DINNER	SNACKS

EXERCISE	REPS	SET -1	SET -2	SET -3	NOTE

TODAY'S FEELINGS	FEELINGS I WANT TO FEEL TOMORROW

DATE: /   /   S   M   T   W   T   F   S

MY DAILY GOALS

MY MOTIVATION

WATER TRACKER

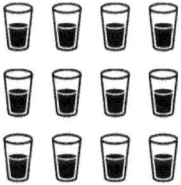

MEALS AND SNACKS

BREAKFAST	LUNCH	DINNER	SNACKS

EXERCISE	REPS	SET -1	SET -2	SET -3	NOTE

TODAY'S FEELINGS	FEELINGS I WANT TO FEEL TOMORROW

DATE: /   /   S   M   T   W   T   F   S

MY DAILY GOALS

MY MOTIVATION

WATER TRACKER

MEALS AND SNACKS

BREAKFAST	LUNCH	DINNER	SNACKS

EXERCISE	REPS	SET -1	SET -2	SET -3	NOTE

TODAY'S FEELINGS	FEELINGS I WANT TO FEEL TOMORROW

DATE: /   /   S   M   T   W   T   F   S

MY DAILY GOALS

WATER
TRACKER

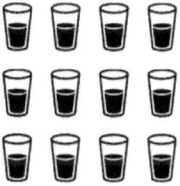

MEALS AND SNACKS

BREAKFAST	LUNCH	DINNER	SNACKS

EXERCISE	REPS	SET -1	SET -2	SET -3	NOTE

TODAY'S FEELINGS

FEELINGS I WANT TO
FEEL TOMORROW

DATE: /   /   S   M   T   W   T   F   S

MY DAILY GOALS

MY MOTIVATION

WATER TRACKER

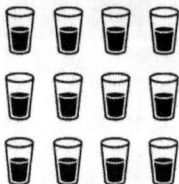

MEALS AND SNACKS

BREAKFAST	LUNCH	DINNER	SNACKS

EXERCISE	REPS	SET -1	SET -2	SET -3	NOTE

TODAY'S FEELINGS	FEELINGS I WANT TO FEEL TOMORROW

DATE: /   /   S   M   T   W   T   F   S

MY DAILY GOALS

MY MOTIVATION

WATER TRACKER

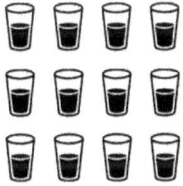

MEALS AND SNACKS

BREAKFAST	LUNCH	DINNER	SNACKS

EXERCISE	REPS	SET -1	SET -2	SET -3	NOTE

TODAY'S FEELINGS	FEELINGS I WANT TO FEEL TOMORROW

DATE: / /   S   M   T   W   T   F   S

MY DAILY GOALS

MY MOTIVATION

WATER TRACKER

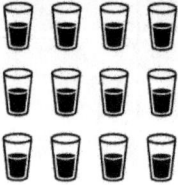

MEALS AND SNACKS

BREAKFAST	LUNCH	DINNER	SNACKS

EXERCISE	REPS	SET -1	SET -2	SET -3	NOTE

TODAY'S FEELINGS	FEELINGS I WANT TO FEEL TOMORROW

DATE: /   /   S   M   T   W   T   F   S

MY DAILY GOALS

MY MOTIVATION

WATER TRACKER

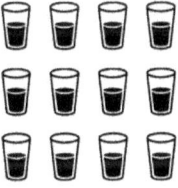

MEALS AND SNACKS

BREAKFAST	LUNCH	DINNER	SNACKS

EXERCISE	REPS	SET -1	SET -2	SET -3	NOTE

TODAY'S FEELINGS	FEELINGS I WANT TO FEEL TOMORROW

DATE: /   /   S   M   T   W   T   F   S

MY DAILY GOALS

MY MOTIVATION

WATER TRACKER

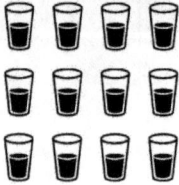

MEALS AND SNACKS

BREAKFAST	LUNCH	DINNER	SNACKS

EXERCISE	REPS	SET -1	SET -2	SET -3	NOTE

TODAY'S FEELINGS	FEELINGS I WANT TO FEEL TOMORROW

DATE: /   /   S   M   T   W   T   F   S

MY DAILY GOALS

MY MOTIVATION

WATER TRACKER

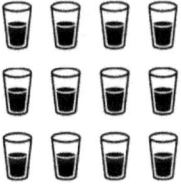

MEALS AND SNACKS

Breakfast	Lunch	Dinner	Snacks

Exercise	Reps	Set -1	Set -2	Set -3	Note

TODAY'S FEELINGS	FEELINGS I WANT TO FEEL TOMORROW

DATE: / /   S   M   T   W   T   F   S

MY DAILY GOALS

MY MOTIVATION

WATER TRACKER

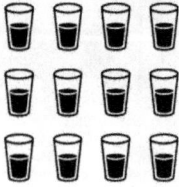

MEALS AND SNACKS

Breakfast	Lunch	Dinner	Snacks

Exercise	Reps	Set -1	Set -2	Set -3	Note

TODAY'S FEELINGS	FEELINGS I WANT TO FEEL TOMORROW

DATE: /   /   S   M   T   W   T   F   S

MY DAILY GOALS

WATER TRACKER

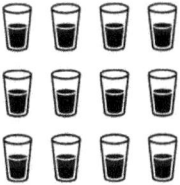

MEALS AND SNACKS

BREAKFAST	LUNCH	DINNER	SNACKS

EXERCISE	REPS	SET -1	SET -2	SET -3	NOTE

TODAY'S FEELINGS	FEELINGS I WANT TO FEEL TOMORROW

DATE: /   /   S   M   T   W   T   F   S

MY DAILY GOALS

MY MOTIVATION

WATER TRACKER

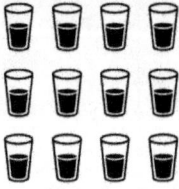

MEALS AND SNACKS

BREAKFAST	LUNCH	DINNER	SNACKS

EXERCISE	REPS	SET -1	SET -2	SET -3	NOTE

TODAY'S FEELINGS	FEELINGS I WANT TO FEEL TOMORROW

DATE: /   /   S   M   T   W   T   F   S

MY DAILY GOALS

MY MOTIVATION

WATER TRACKER

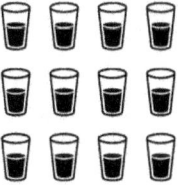

MEALS AND SNACKS

BREAKFAST	LUNCH	DINNER	SNACKS

EXERCISE	REPS	SET -1	SET -2	SET -3	NOTE

TODAY'S FEELINGS	FEELINGS I WANT TO FEEL TOMORROW

DATE: / /   S   M   T   W   T   F   S

MY DAILY GOALS

MY MOTIVATION

WATER TRACKER

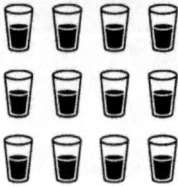

MEALS AND SNACKS

BREAKFAST	LUNCH	DINNER	SNACKS

EXERCISE	REPS	SET -1	SET -2	SET -3	NOTE

TODAY'S FEELINGS	FEELINGS I WANT TO FEEL TOMORROW

DATE: / /   S   M   T   W   T   F   S

MY DAILY GOALS

MY MOTIVATION

WATER TRACKER

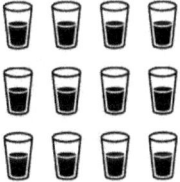

MEALS AND SNACKS

BREAKFAST	LUNCH	DINNER	SNACKS

EXERCISE	REPS	SET -1	SET -2	SET -3	NOTE

TODAY'S FEELINGS	FEELINGS I WANT TO FEEL TOMORROW

DATE: / / S M T W T F S

MY DAILY GOALS

MY MOTIVATION

WATER TRACKER

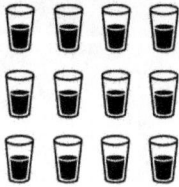

MEALS AND SNACKS

BREAKFAST	LUNCH	DINNER	SNACKS

EXERCISE	REPS	SET -1	SET -2	SET -3	NOTE

TODAY'S FEELINGS	FEELINGS I WANT TO FEEL TOMORROW

DATE: / /   S   M   T   W   T   F   S

MY DAILY GOALS

MY MOTIVATION

WATER TRACKER

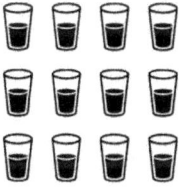

MEALS AND SNACKS

BREAKFAST	LUNCH	DINNER	SNACKS

EXERCISE	REPS	SET -1	SET -2	SET -3	NOTE

TODAY'S FEELINGS	FEELINGS I WANT TO FEEL TOMORROW

DATE: /   /   S   M   T   W   T   F   S

MY DAILY GOALS

WATER TRACKER

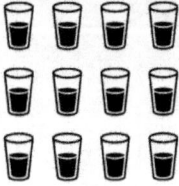

MEALS AND SNACKS

BREAKFAST	LUNCH	DINNER	SNACKS

EXERCISE	REPS	SET -1	SET -2	SET -3	NOTE

TODAY'S FEELINGS	FEELINGS I WANT TO FEEL TOMORROW

DATE: / / S M T W T F S

MY DAILY GOALS

MY MOTIVATION

WATER TRACKER

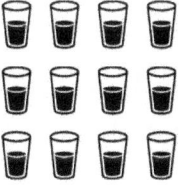

MEALS AND SNACKS

BREAKFAST	LUNCH	DINNER	SNACKS

EXERCISE	REPS	SET -1	SET -2	SET -3	NOTE

TODAY'S FEELINGS

FEELINGS I WANT TO FEEL TOMORROW

DATE: / /   S M T W T F S

MY DAILY GOALS

MY MOTIVATION

WATER TRACKER

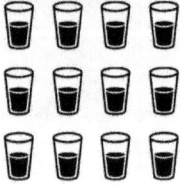

MEALS AND SNACKS

BREAKFAST	LUNCH	DINNER	SNACKS

EXERCISE	REPS	SET -1	SET -2	SET -3	NOTE

TODAY'S FEELINGS	FEELINGS I WANT TO FEEL TOMORROW

DATE: /   /   S   M   T   W   T   F   S

MY DAILY GOALS

WATER
TRACKER

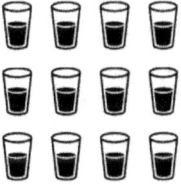

MEALS AND SNACKS

BREAKFAST	LUNCH	DINNER	SNACKS

EXERCISE	REPS	SET -1	SET -2	SET -3	NOTE

TODAY'S FEELINGS	FEELINGS I WANT TO FEEL TOMORROW

DATE: /   /   S   M   T   W   T   F   S

MY DAILY GOALS

MY MOTIVATION

WATER TRACKER

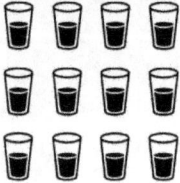

MEALS AND SNACKS

BREAKFAST	LUNCH	DINNER	SNACKS

EXERCISE	REPS	SET -1	SET -2	SET -3	NOTE

TODAY'S FEELINGS	FEELINGS I WANT TO FEEL TOMORROW

DATE: /   /   S   M   T   W   T   F   S

MY DAILY GOALS   MY MOTIVATION

WATER
TRACKER   MEALS AND SNACKS

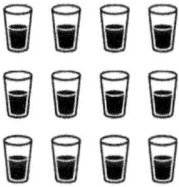

	BREAKFAST	LUNCH	DINNER	SNACKS

EXERCISE	REPS	SET -1	SET -2	SET -3	NOTE

TODAY'S FEELINGS   FEELINGS I WANT TO
                                 FEEL TOMORROW

DATE: / /   S M T W T F S

MY DAILY GOALS

MY MOTIVATION

WATER
TRACKER

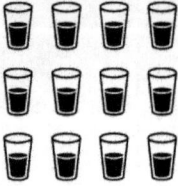

MEALS AND SNACKS

BREAKFAST	LUNCH	DINNER	SNACKS

EXERCISE	REPS	SET -1	SET -2	SET -3	NOTE

TODAY'S FEELINGS	FEELINGS I WANT TO FEEL TOMORROW

DATE: /   /   S   M   T   W   T   F   S

MY DAILY GOALS

MY MOTIVATION

WATER TRACKER

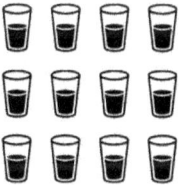

MEALS AND SNACKS

BREAKFAST	LUNCH	DINNER	SNACKS

EXERCISE	REPS	SET -1	SET -2	SET -3	NOTE

TODAY'S FEELINGS	FEELINGS I WANT TO FEEL TOMORROW

DATE: / / S M T W T F S

MY DAILY GOALS

MY MOTIVATION

WATER TRACKER

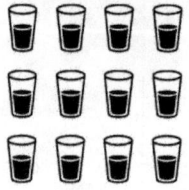

MEALS AND SNACKS

BREAKFAST	LUNCH	DINNER	SNACKS

EXERCISE	REPS	SET -1	SET -2	SET -3	NOTE

TODAY'S FEELINGS	FEELINGS I WANT TO FEEL TOMORROW

DATE: /   /   S   M   T   W   T   F   S

MY DAILY GOALS

MY MOTIVATION

WATER
TRACKER

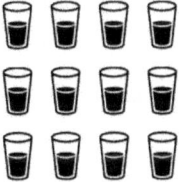

MEALS AND SNACKS

BREAKFAST	LUNCH	DINNER	SNACKS

EXERCISE	REPS	SET -1	SET -2	SET -3	NOTE

TODAY'S FEELINGS	FEELINGS I WANT TO FEEL TOMORROW

DATE: /   /   S   M   T   W   T   F   S

MY DAILY GOALS

MY MOTIVATION

WATER TRACKER

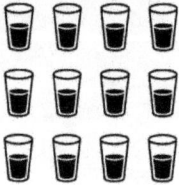

MEALS AND SNACKS

BREAKFAST	LUNCH	DINNER	SNACKS

EXERCISE	REPS	SET -1	SET -2	SET -3	NOTE

TODAY'S FEELINGS	FEELINGS I WANT TO FEEL TOMORROW

DATE: /   /   S   M   T   W   T   F   S

MY DAILY GOALS

MY MOTIVATION

WATER TRACKER

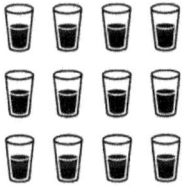

MEALS AND SNACKS

BREAKFAST	LUNCH	DINNER	SNACKS

EXERCISE	REPS	SET -1	SET -2	SET -3	NOTE

TODAY'S FEELINGS

FEELINGS I WANT TO FEEL TOMORROW

DATE: /   /   S   M   T   W   T   F   S

MY DAILY GOALS

WATER TRACKER

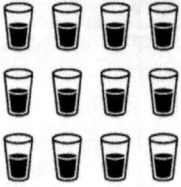

MEALS AND SNACKS

BREAKFAST	LUNCH	DINNER	SNACKS

EXERCISE	REPS	SET -1	SET -2	SET -3	NOTE

TODAY'S FEELINGS	FEELINGS I WANT TO FEEL TOMORROW

DATE: / /   S M T W T F S

MY DAILY GOALS

MY MOTIVATION

WATER TRACKER

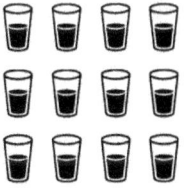

MEALS AND SNACKS

BREAKFAST	LUNCH	DINNER	SNACKS

EXERCISE	REPS	SET -1	SET -2	SET -3	NOTE

TODAY'S FEELINGS	FEELINGS I WANT TO FEEL TOMORROW

DATE: / /   S M T W T F S

MY DAILY GOALS

MY MOTIVATION

WATER TRACKER

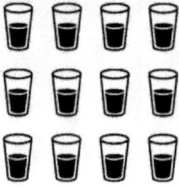

MEALS AND SNACKS

BREAKFAST	LUNCH	DINNER	SNACKS

EXERCISE	REPS	SET -1	SET -2	SET -3	NOTE

TODAY'S FEELINGS

FEELINGS I WANT TO FEEL TOMORROW

DATE: /   /   S   M   T   W   T   F   S

MY DAILY GOALS

MY MOTIVATION

WATER TRACKER

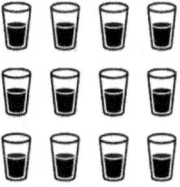

MEALS AND SNACKS

BREAKFAST	LUNCH	DINNER	SNACKS

EXERCISE	REPS	SET -1	SET -2	SET -3	NOTE

TODAY'S FEELINGS	FEELINGS I WANT TO FEEL TOMORROW

DATE: / /   S M T W T F S

MY DAILY GOALS

WATER TRACKER

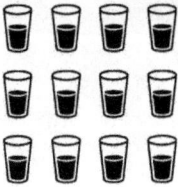

MEALS AND SNACKS

BREAKFAST	LUNCH	DINNER	SNACKS

EXERCISE	REPS	SET -1	SET -2	SET -3	NOTE

TODAY'S FEELINGS	FEELINGS I WANT TO FEEL TOMORROW

DATE: /   /   S   M   T   W   T   F   S

MY DAILY GOALS

MY MOTIVATION

WATER TRACKER

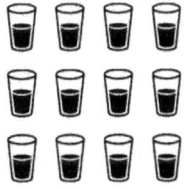

MEALS AND SNACKS

BREAKFAST	LUNCH	DINNER	SNACKS

EXERCISE	REPS	SET -1	SET -2	SET -3	NOTE

TODAY'S FEELINGS	FEELINGS I WANT TO FEEL TOMORROW

DATE: /   /   S   M   T   W   T   F   S

MY DAILY GOALS

MY MOTIVATION

WATER TRACKER

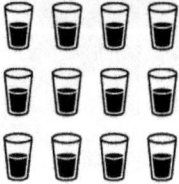

MEALS AND SNACKS

BREAKFAST	LUNCH	DINNER	SNACKS

EXERCISE	REPS	SET -1	SET -2	SET -3	NOTE

TODAY'S FEELINGS

FEELINGS I WANT TO FEEL TOMORROW

DATE: / /   S   M   T   W   T   F   S

MY DAILY GOALS

MY MOTIVATION

WATER TRACKER

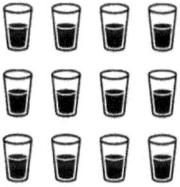

MEALS AND SNACKS

BREAKFAST	LUNCH	DINNER	SNACKS

EXERCISE	REPS	SET -1	SET -2	SET -3	NOTE

TODAY'S FEELINGS	FEELINGS I WANT TO FEEL TOMORROW

DATE: / /   S M T W T F S

MY DAILY GOALS

WATER TRACKER

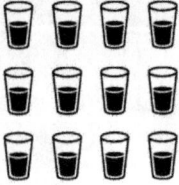

MEALS AND SNACKS

BREAKFAST	LUNCH	DINNER	SNACKS

EXERCISE	REPS	SET -1	SET -2	SET -3	NOTE

TODAY'S FEELINGS	FEELINGS I WANT TO FEEL TOMORROW

DATE: / / S M T W T F S

MY DAILY GOALS

MY MOTIVATION

WATER TRACKER

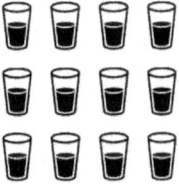

MEALS AND SNACKS

BREAKFAST	LUNCH	DINNER	SNACKS

EXERCISE	REPS	SET -1	SET -2	SET -3	NOTE

TODAY'S FEELINGS	FEELINGS I WANT TO FEEL TOMORROW

DATE: /   /   S   M   T   W   T   F   S

MY DAILY GOALS

MY MOTIVATION

WATER TRACKER

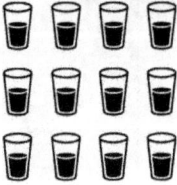

MEALS AND SNACKS

BREAKFAST	LUNCH	DINNER	SNACKS

EXERCISE	REPS	SET -1	SET -2	SET -3	NOTE

TODAY'S FEELINGS	FEELINGS I WANT TO FEEL TOMORROW

DATE: / /   S M T W T F S

MY DAILY GOALS

WATER TRACKER	MEALS AND SNACKS			
	BREAKFAST	LUNCH	DINNER	SNACKS

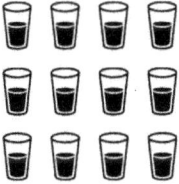

EXERCISE	REPS	SET -1	SET -2	SET -3	NOTE

TODAY'S FEELINGS	FEELINGS I WANT TO FEEL TOMORROW

DATE: /   /   S   M   T   W   T   F   S

MY DAILY GOALS

MY MOTIVATION

WATER TRACKER

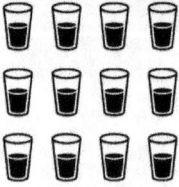

MEALS AND SNACKS

BREAKFAST	LUNCH	DINNER	SNACKS

EXERCISE	REPS	SET -1	SET -2	SET -3	NOTE

TODAY'S FEELINGS	FEELINGS I WANT TO FEEL TOMORROW

DATE: /   /   S   M   T   W   T   F   S

MY DAILY GOALS

MY MOTIVATION

WATER TRACKER

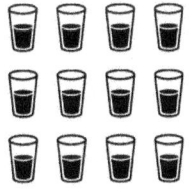

MEALS AND SNACKS

BREAKFAST	LUNCH	DINNER	SNACKS

EXERCISE	REPS	SET -1	SET -2	SET -3	NOTE

TODAY'S FEELINGS	FEELINGS I WANT TO FEEL TOMORROW

DATE: / /   S M T W T F S

MY DAILY GOALS

MY MOTIVATION

WATER TRACKER

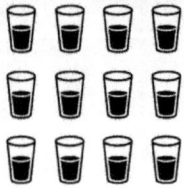

MEALS AND SNACKS

BREAKFAST	LUNCH	DINNER	SNACKS

EXERCISE	REPS	SET -1	SET -2	SET -3	NOTE

TODAY'S FEELINGS

FEELINGS I WANT TO FEEL TOMORROW

DATE: /   /   S   M   T   W   T   F   S

MY DAILY GOALS

MY MOTIVATION

WATER TRACKER

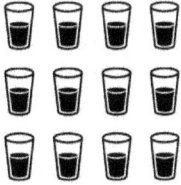

MEALS AND SNACKS

BREAKFAST	LUNCH	DINNER	SNACKS

EXERCISE	REPS	SET -1	SET -2	SET -3	NOTE

TODAY'S FEELINGS	FEELINGS I WANT TO FEEL TOMORROW

DATE: /   /   S   M   T   W   T   F   S

MY DAILY GOALS

MY MOTIVATION

WATER TRACKER

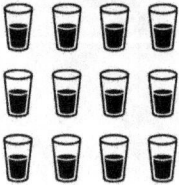

MEALS AND SNACKS

Breakfast	Lunch	Dinner	Snacks

Exercise	Reps	Set -1	Set -2	Set -3	Note

TODAY'S FEELINGS	FEELINGS I WANT TO FEEL TOMORROW

DATE: / /   S M T W T F S

MY DAILY GOALS

MY MOTIVATION

WATER TRACKER

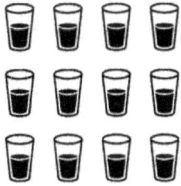

MEALS AND SNACKS

BREAKFAST	LUNCH	DINNER	SNACKS

EXERCISE	REPS	SET -1	SET -2	SET -3	NOTE

TODAY'S FEELINGS

FEELINGS I WANT TO FEEL TOMORROW

DATE: /   /   S   M   T   W   T   F   S

MY DAILY GOALS

MY MOTIVATION

WATER TRACKER

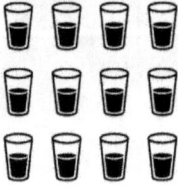

MEALS AND SNACKS

BREAKFAST	LUNCH	DINNER	SNACKS

EXERCISE	REPS	SET -1	SET -2	SET -3	NOTE

TODAY'S FEELINGS

FEELINGS I WANT TO FEEL TOMORROW

DATE: /   /   S   M   T   W   T   F   S

MY DAILY GOALS

WATER
TRACKER

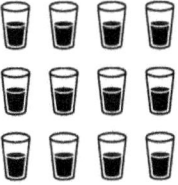

MEALS AND SNACKS

BREAKFAST	LUNCH	DINNER	SNACKS

EXERCISE	REPS	SET -1	SET -2	SET -3	NOTE

TODAY'S FEELINGS	FEELINGS I WANT TO FEEL TOMORROW

DATE: /   /   S   M   T   W   T   F   S

MY DAILY GOALS

MY MOTIVATION

WATER TRACKER

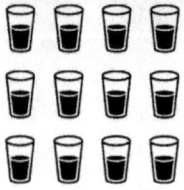

MEALS AND SNACKS

BREAKFAST	LUNCH	DINNER	SNACKS

EXERCISE	REPS	SET -1	SET -2	SET -3	NOTE

TODAY'S FEELINGS	FEELINGS I WANT TO FEEL TOMORROW

DATE: /   /   S   M   T   W   T   F   S

MY DAILY GOALS

MY MOTIVATION

WATER TRACKER

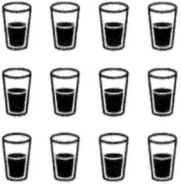

MEALS AND SNACKS

BREAKFAST	LUNCH	DINNER	SNACKS

EXERCISE	REPS	SET -1	SET -2	SET -3	NOTE

TODAY'S FEELINGS	FEELINGS I WANT TO FEEL TOMORROW

NOTES

Date :　　/　　/

NOTES

Date : / /

NOTES

Date :   /   /

NOTES

Date :   /   /

NOTES

Date :   /   /

NOTES

Date : / /

NOTES

Date :   /   /

NOTES

Date: / /

NOTES

Date :   /   /

NOTES

Date: / /

BODY MEASUREMENT

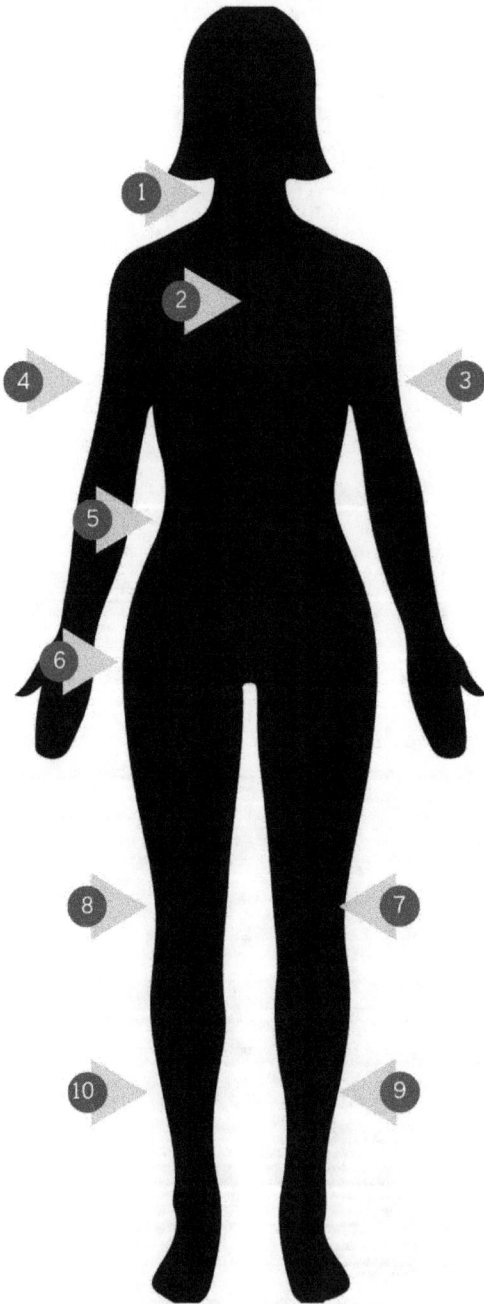

		AFTER
DATE:		
WEIGHT:		
1	NECK	
2	CHEST	
3	LEFT ARM	
4	RIGHT ARM	
5	WAIST	
6	HIPS	
7	LEFT THIGH	
8	RIGHT THIGH	
9	LEFT CALF:	
10	RIGHT CALF